ShanShan Yoga

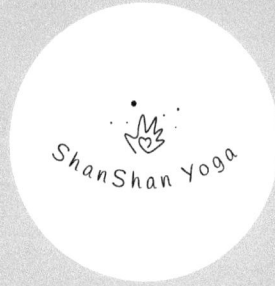

Yoga at Your Desk

A practical guide for short breaks during your working day.

SHANI ABERGIL

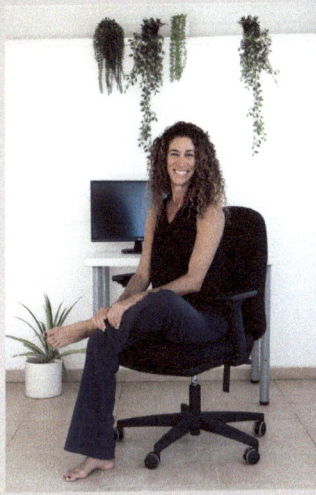

Shani is a Yoga therapist with a passion for helping people find balance and well-being through a personalized, holistic approach to health.

She has been teaching Yoga to individuals and groups since 2009, and believes that a genuine smile during practice brings peace and spreads joy to those around us.

Drawing on over two decades of experience in the IT industry, she combines delivery leadership with mindfulness to help professionals navigate stress, strengthen focus, and nurture balance within fast-paced company cultures.

YOGA@SHANSHAN.COM.AU

CONTENTS

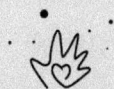

1

BREATHE

Breath is a powerful anchor, helping to steady the mind and reconnect you to the present moment.

By lengthening and balancing inhalations and exhalations, breath awareness improves oxygen exchange, supports healthy circulation, and enhances focus and clarity.

Bringing mindful attention to the breath helps calm the nervous system and reduce stress, creating a greater sense of ease in both body and mind.

Taking just a few minutes between meetings to notice your breath can help restore calm and focus.

Throughout this book I recommend closing the eyes and smiling. Allowing a slight smile not only eases the muscles of the face but also encourages a state of openness and positivity throughout the body.

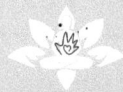

Exercise 1: Breath awareness

Begin by sitting forward on your chair with your feet firmly planted on the floor. Rest your hands on your thighs or place one hand on the belly and one on the chest. Allow your spine to lengthen, gently tuck your chin in, imagining a line extending from your tailbone to the crown of your head.

You may keep your gaze soft and forward, or close your eyes to rest from outside distractions. Breathe slowly in and out through your nose, observing the natural rhythm of your breath as it moves through your body.

On each inhalation, feel the belly rise, followed by the expansion of the ribs and chest. On each exhalation, notice the release from the belly, lungs, and chest. Continue to follow this wave-like movement of breath, cultivating awareness with every cycle.

With your breath, invite nourishment into your body and mind. Inhale a sense of vitality into every cell, and exhale any tension you may be holding.

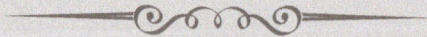

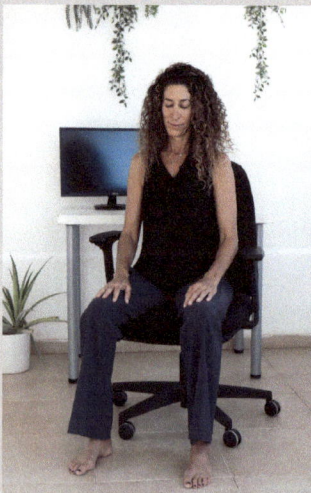

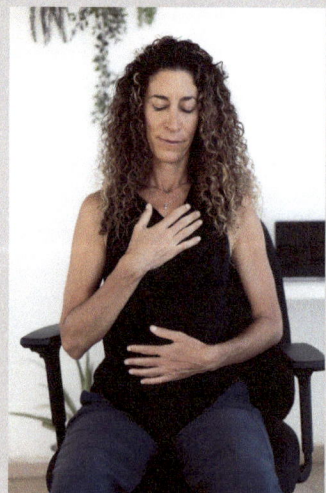

Exercise 2: Extended exhalation

Sit forward on your chair with your feet firmly on the floor and your spine elongated. Rest your hands on your thighs and gently soften your shoulders.

Begin by breathing in and out through your nose. Inhale for a count of four, and exhale for a count of four.

After a few rounds, start to lengthen the exhalation. Inhale for four and exhale for six, keeping the breath smooth and without strain. If comfortable, you may gradually extend the length of the exhalation further, always staying attuned to how you feel in the moment.

When you are ready to finish, bring your palms to rest gently over your eyes. Take a pause here to notice the effects of your practice and to acknowledge the gift of giving yourself a mindful break in the middle of your day.

When you are ready, release your hands, smile, and open your eyes.

2

NECK

The neck muscles have an important role in stimulating the vagus nerve - promoting stress reduction and boosting our immune system.

When the neck becomes tense from stress, poor posture, or long hours at a desk, this tension can restrict mobility, contribute to headaches, and disrupt the natural balance of the nervous system.

Gentle neck releases not only help ease physical tightness but also create space for freer breathing and improved circulation. By combining these releases with mindful nerve gliding exercises, we can restore healthy movement along the nerves that pass through the neck and shoulders, reduce discomfort, and support overall relaxation.

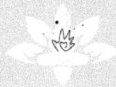

Exercise 1: Side neck stretch

Sit forward on your chair with an elongated spine. Make sure your feet are on the ground, hip width distance. Extend your arms to the side (about 45 degrees), reaching through the fingers, shoulders relaxed and freed of tension (soft).

Slowly bring your right ear toward your right shoulder. Go to where it feels slightly stretched - stay and breath. Mindfully soften both shoulders and keep stretching through your fingers. Closing your eyes while in the posture helps connecting to the sensations. After 5-8 breaths, return to centre and change sides.

Optional - Gentle half-circle neck movements

Transition between sides with a smooth half-circle motion, guiding your chin toward your chest.

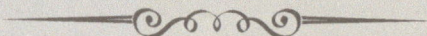

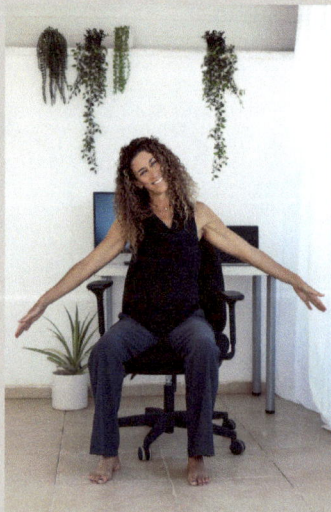

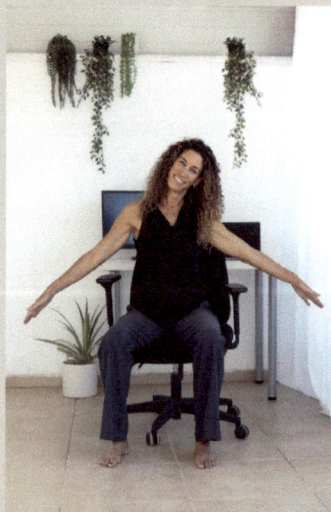

Nerve gliding

Nerve gliding (or neurodynamic) exercises gently mobilize nerves through their natural pathways. They are often used to:
- Reduce nerve-related tension or discomfort (like tingling, numbness, or radiating pain)
- Improve mobility and nerve health
- Support recovery from issues like cervical radiculopathy, carpal tunnel, or thoracic outlet syndrome.

They differ from stretches: instead of lengthening a muscle, you're gliding the nerve back and forth within its sheath to reduce irritation or compression.

Important Notes for nerve gliding exercises:
- These should be pain-free — a light tingling is okay, sharpness or increased symptoms is not.
- Movements are gentle and controlled, like "flossing" the nerve through tissue.
- In case of a known nerve damage, please avoid the next few exercises.

Exercise 1: Median nerve glide

The median nerve runs from the neck down the front of the arm into the hand, and it controls sensation and movement in the thumb, index, and middle fingers, playing a key role in grip and fine motor skills.

The purpose of the Median Nerve Glide is to release tension and improve mobility through the front of the arm and hand.

Sit upright and relax your shoulders. Extend one arm out to the side at shoulder height, palm facing up. Gently bend your wrist back (fingers pointing up). Slowly tilt your head away from the extended arm. Hold for a few breaths, smile.

Return to center, and repeat on the other side.

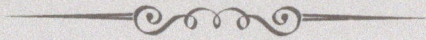

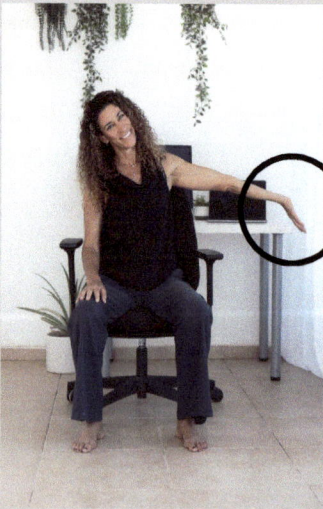

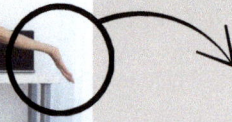

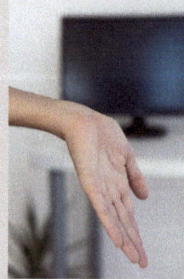

Exercise 2: Ulnar nerve glide

The ulnar nerve travels from the neck down the inner arm to the ring and little fingers, and it helps control fine motor movement in the hand and provides sensation to the outer edge of the hand and fingers.

The purpose of the Ulnar Nerve Glide is to ease strain along the inner elbow, wrist, and hand.

Sit tall and extend both arms out to the side like a letter "T". Bend your elbows slightly and turn your palms up. Let your wrists drop gently (fingers point toward the ceiling).
Slowly extend one arm to the side, fingers facing up. If comfortable, start to tilt your head away from the extended arm, hold, smile, then return to center.

Repeat on the other side.

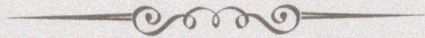

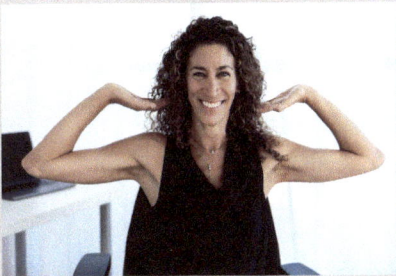

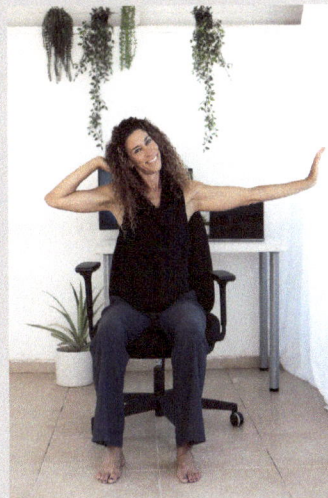

Exercise 3: Radial nerve glide

The radial nerve runs along the back of the arm and forearm, and it controls extension of the wrist and fingers, as well as sensation to the back of the hand and thumb side.

The purpose of the Radial Nerve Glide is to relieve tension from the shoulder to the back of the hand.

Sit tall and extend one arm slightly behind your body with the palm facing down. Connect your thumb add index finger, bring fingers towards the wrist and turn the hand upwards towards the ceiling.
Tilt your head to the opposite side, feeling a light tension.
Stay for several breaths. Smile.

Return to center and repeat on the other side.

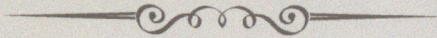

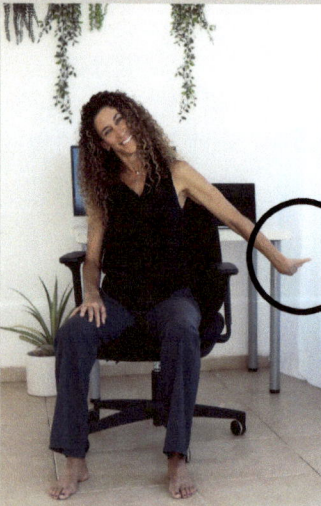

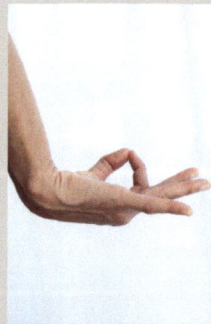

3

TWIST IT

Seated twists offer a wide range of benefits for both the body and mind.

Physically, they help improve spinal mobility, support healthy posture, and release tension through the back, shoulders, and neck. By gently compressing and releasing the abdominal area, twists also stimulate digestion and encourage better circulation through the core.

Practising seated twists promotes mindful breathing, creating space between the vertebrae and inviting a sense of lightness and ease.

Emotionally, twists can help release stored tension, offering a refreshing sense of reset and balance throughout the body.

It is recommended that you twist on an empty stomach, but gentle twists can be done at any time.

Exercise 1: Active seated twist

Sit forward on your chair with an elongated spine and your feet grounded on the floor. Raise your arms to the side, shoulders height. Bend your elbows with the palms facing up.

On your inhalation, allow your spine to grow tall. As you start to exhale - twist to your right side. Lead the movement with your elbows, keeping the sitting bones firmly on the chair. Inhale to come back to the centre and, on your exhale, twist to your left side. Continue the dynamic twists on each side and on the third cycle stay in the twist for 3-5 breaths in each side.

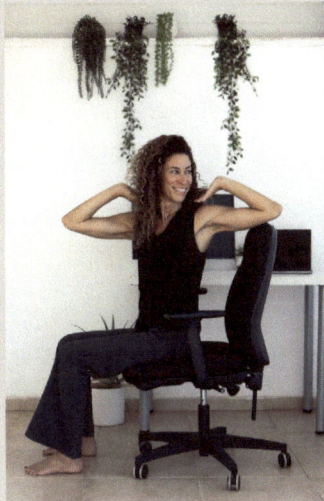

When you come back to the centre ,let your hands rest on your thighs, close your eyes for a moment and feel the sensations in your body. Smile.

Exercise 2: Deep seated twist

Sitting for long periods can place pressure on the lower back. This variation of a seated twist offers gentle release and support for that area.

Sit forward on your chair and bring your hands together in a prayer position. Tilt your body forward and begin to twist to the right. If available, bring your elbow to the outside of the opposite thigh to deepen the twist. Alternatively, you may open your arms and use the back of your arm as gentle leverage. Allow your gaze to remain to the side or, if comfortable, turn your head upward.

As you hold the twist, encourage long, steady breaths, noticing the belly meeting the thigh with each inhalation and exhalation. Stay for 3–5 breaths before slowly returning upright.

Repeat on the other side.

When you return to the centre, rest your hands on your thighs, close your eyes and smile.

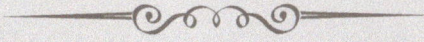

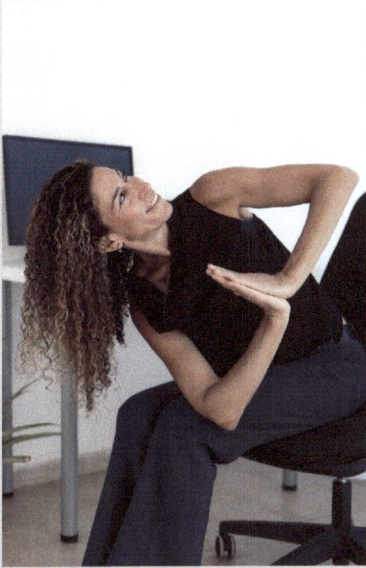

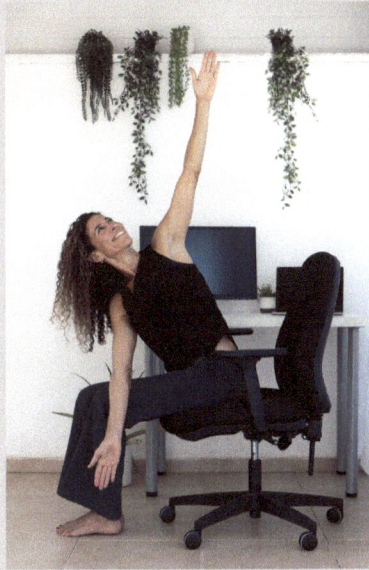

SHOULDERS 4

The shoulders play an important role in our physical, psychological, and even spiritual well-being.

Physically, they are vital for arm mobility and strength, supported by muscles such as the deltoids, trapezius, and rotator cuff, which stabilize and move the shoulder joint.

Psychologically, shoulders often symbolize strength and resilience. Our posture and the way we carry them can express confidence or vulnerability. They also represent responsibility — the weight of duties we "carry on our shoulders" — and provide a sense of protection and support.

Spiritually, the shoulders are seen as channels for energy flow and as common areas where emotional tension accumulates. Practices such as yoga, massage, and mindful movement help release this tension and restore balance.

When working at a desk or computer, the shoulders often bear the burden of poor posture. The following exercises focus on releasing tightness and strengthening the shoulder joints for better alignment and ease.

Exercise 1: Shoulders' mobility

Sit tall on your chair with your spine elongated and feet grounded on the floor. Bend your arms to 90 degrees and lift your elbows to shoulder height.

On an inhalation, draw the elbows back to a comfortable range, squeezing the shoulder blades together to open the chest. As you exhale, bring the elbows and forearms toward one another in front of the chest. Continue in this rhythm - inhale to open and expand, exhale to close and release.

Repeat for several breaths. Smile.

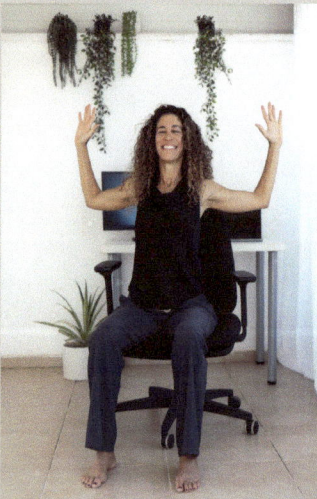

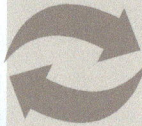

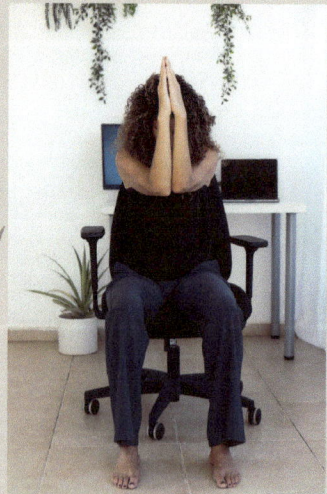

Optional – Add spinal movements

To add spinal movement, inhale as you arch the back and lift the chest, allowing the gaze to rise if the neck feels comfortable. Exhale as you round the back, bringing the chin gently toward the chest as the elbows come together.

Repeat th sequence for several breaths.

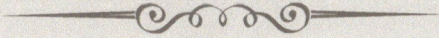

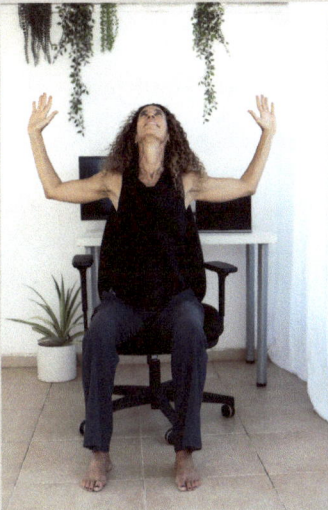

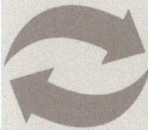

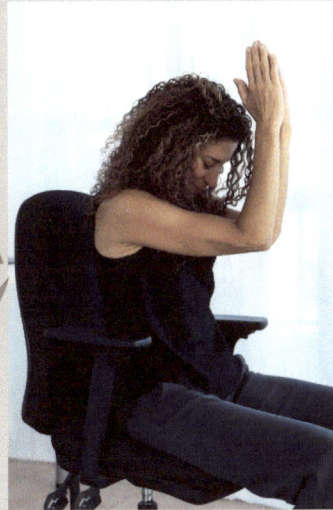

Exercise 2: Shoulders' flexibility

For this exercise you will need a resistance band, a scarf or a belt. I am using a scarf for the examples bellow.

Hold the scarf with your arms extended straight out in front of you at shoulder height. Make sure the scarf is taut but not overly stretched.
Keeping your arms straight, begin by slowly raising your arms overhead, bringing the scarf up and over your head as you inhale, and lower the arms as you exhale. Continue for 3 breaths.

On your next inhale, bring your arms up overhead and exhale to lower to the right side. Inhale, return to overhead position, and exhale to the left side. Continue for 3 breaths.

From your arms overhead position, slowly start to take the arms back behind you as you exhale. If you need to bend your elbows, widen your hold on the scarf. On your inhale bring your arms back overheard. Continue for 3 breaths. Smile.

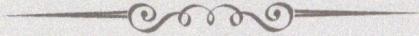

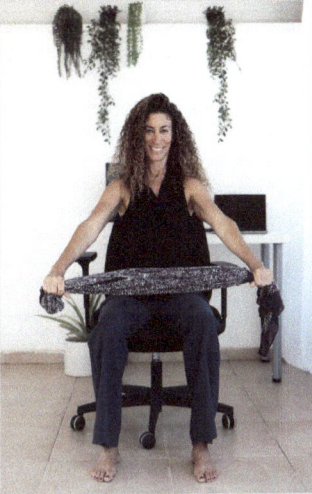 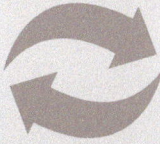 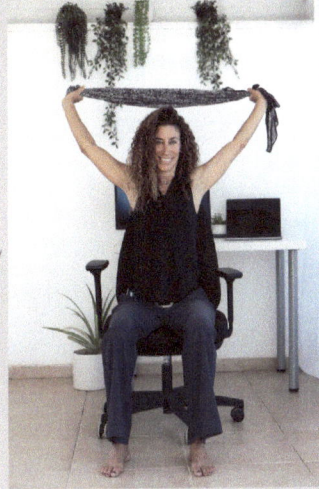

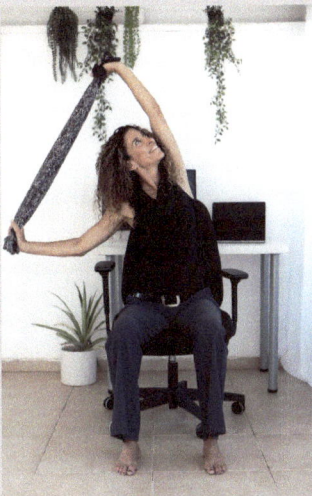 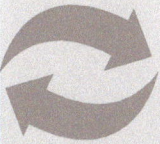 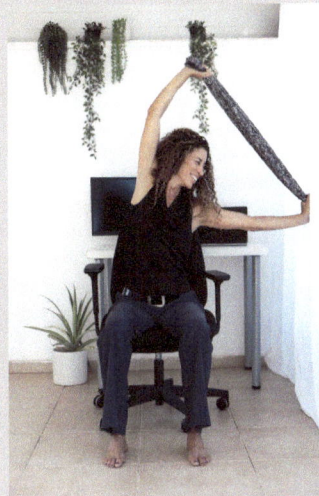

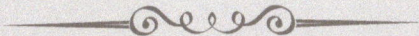

For most of us, taking the arms back behind us is difficult as we tend to close the chest when working in front of our computer screens.

For the next few breaths, find the position in which you felt it the most and stay there.

Keep breathing into the areas you feel need the most attention and allow this tension to fold away as you exhale and smile.

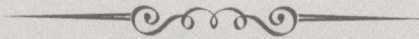

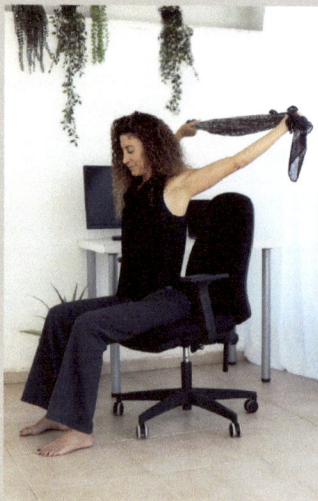

Exercise 3: Shoulders' stretch

This stretch primarily targets the shoulder muscles, including the deltoids and rotator cuff muscles.

This exercise can be done sitting or standing. Hold the ends of the scarf in each hand. Lift your right arm straight overhead, bending it at the elbow so your hand is positioned behind your head, palm facing down. Reach your left hand behind your back and grab the bottom end of the scarf.

Gently pull down on the bottom end of the scarf with your left hand, while simultaneously pulling up on the top end with your right hand. This action will create a gentle stretch along the outside of your right shoulder and arm. Keep your shoulders relaxed and avoid shrugging.

Hold the stretch for 15-30 seconds, focusing on deep breathing and smile to help relax the muscles.

Repeat on the other side.

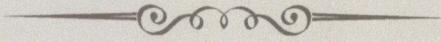

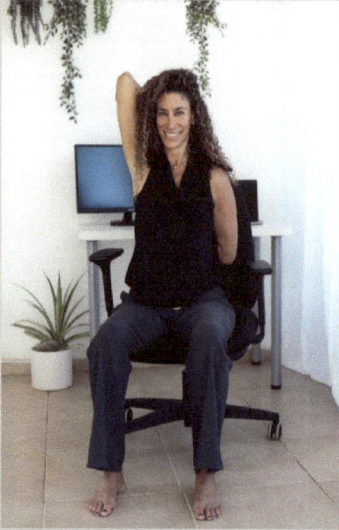

Keep walking the
hands toward one
another.

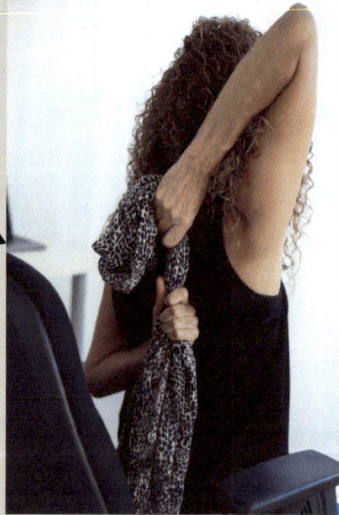

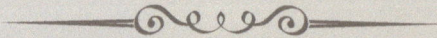

5
FINGERS & WRISTS

Spending long hours at a computer can put strain on the wrists and fingers. Gentle strengthening and flexibility exercises offer several important benefits:

- **Reduced Risk of Strain**: Regular movement helps prevent conditions such as carpal tunnel, tendonitis, and wrist fatigue.
- **Better Ergonomics**: Stronger wrists support healthier typing and mouse use, improving posture and reducing discomfort.
- **Relief from Tension**: Stretches and exercises ease stiffness, boost circulation, and reduce fatigue from repetitive use.
- **Joint Health**: Keeping the hands mobile promotes joint lubrication and long-term function, reducing risk of arthritis and similar conditions.
- **Stress Relief**: Short movement breaks release muscle tension, calm the mind, and restore focus.

Following are several simple wrists and fingers practices that would help relieve tension and strengthen the joints.

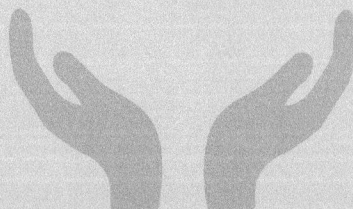

Exercise 1: Wrists rolls

A simple but effective movement to release tension and improve circulation in the hands and wrists is wrist rolls.

Extend your arms above your head, hands relaxed. Slowly start rotating your wrists in large, smooth circles— Ten times in one direction, then ten in the other.

Keep your fingers loose and let the motion come from the wrist joint.

You can repeat with soft fists to add gentle strength and control.

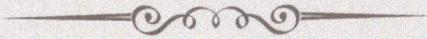

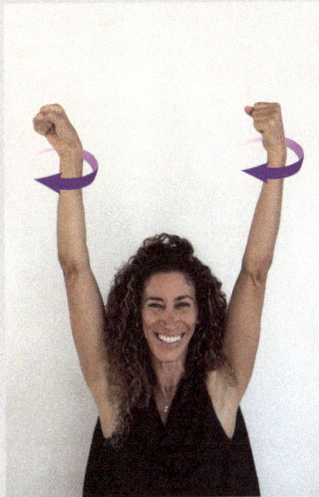

Exercise 2: Wrist extension stretch

To gently stretch the wrists and counteract tightness from everyday use, try the wrist extension stretch.

Extend one arm in front of you with the palm facing up. Use your other hand to gently pull back on the fingers, creating a stretch through the underside of the wrist and forearm.

Hold for 15–30 seconds, then switch sides. Keep the shoulders relaxed and avoid forcing the stretch—this should feel like a release, not a strain.

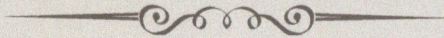

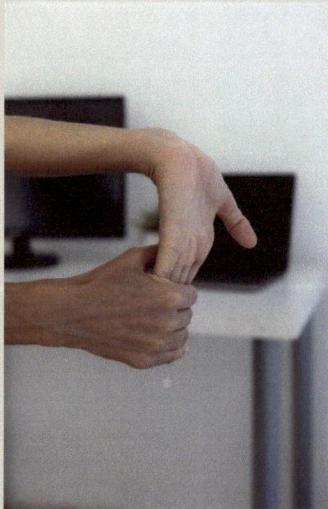

Exercise 3: Fingers stretch and shake

To release stiffness in the fingers and restore mobility, try this quick combination of stretch and movement.

Start by spreading your fingers wide apart, holding the stretch for a few seconds, then make a tight fist. Repeat this open-close motion, you can increase the speed.

Afterward, shake out your hands gently, letting the fingers relax and dangle. This helps reduce built-up tension from gripping, typing, or phone use, and brings fresh blood flow to the smaller joints and muscles. It's a great reset during the day!

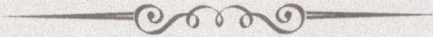

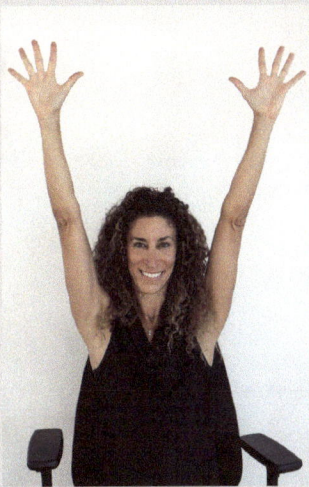

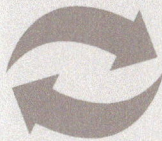

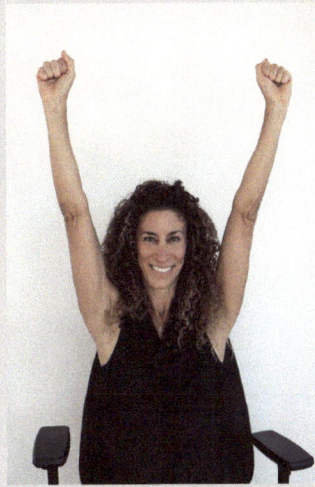

6
SPINAL
MOVEMENTS

Regular spinal movement is essential for maintaining flexibility and preventing stiffness, helping reduce the risk of discomfort or injury.

Engaging in movements that target the spine support healthy posture and alignment, improved balance and coordination.

These movements also encourage circulation and nerve function, nourishing the spinal discs and supporting long-term spinal health. By easing muscular tension around the spine, they promote relaxation and can even uplift your mood!

The following practices can be done as mini breaks while you are sitting in front of your desk.

Exercise 1: Spine mobility – Seated Cat-Cow

To bring gentle motion to the spine and release stiffness from sitting, try seated cat-cow.

Sit upright with your feet grounded and hands resting on your knees. As you inhale, arch your back slightly, lift your chest, and look up—this is your cow pose. As you exhale, round your spine, tuck your chin to your chest, and gently pull your belly in—this is your cat pose.

Move slowly with your breath for 5–10 rounds. You can close your eyes and smile as you move.

This forward-and-back motion helps rehydrate the spinal discs, release tension through the back and neck, and restore spine mobility.

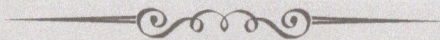

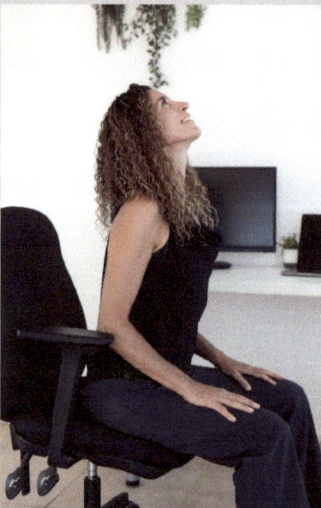

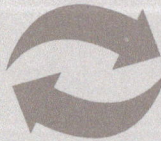

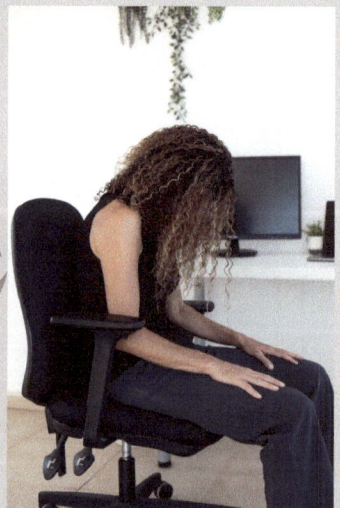

Exercise 2: Spine mobility – Seated Spinal Circles

To loosen up the lower back and pelvis, seated spinal circles are a great choice.

Sit comfortably at the edge of a chair with your hands resting on your knees. Start to slowly circle your torso, shifting your weight forward, then to one side, leaning back slightly, and to the other side—drawing big, smooth circles with your upper body.

Keep the movement relaxed and connected to your breath. Do 5 circles in one direction, then reverse. Smile.

This movement massages the spine, hips, and abdominal organs, while releasing built-up tension from long periods of stillness.

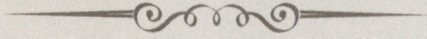

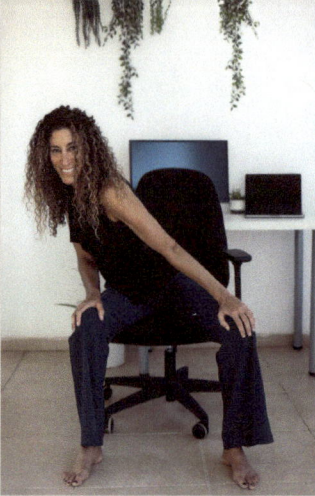

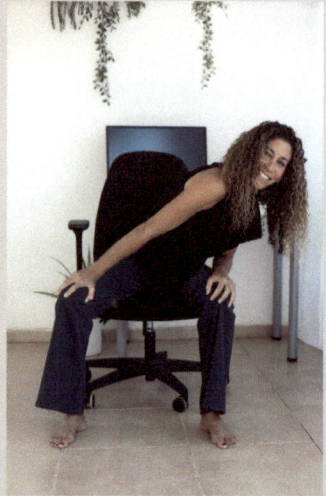

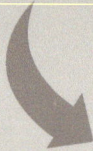

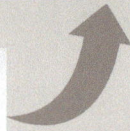

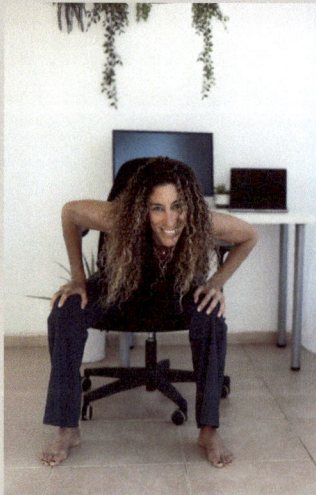

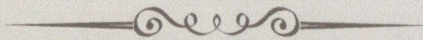

Exercise 3: Seated Spinal Twist

While seated, bring your hands behind your head and interlace your fingers. Open your elbows wide and sit up tall.
Inhale to lengthen the spine. As you exhale, twist through the torso and fold forward, bringing your right elbow toward your left knee.

Inhale to return to center, lifting back up with control. Repeat on the other side.

Move with your breath and keep the core gently engaged to support the spine.

This dynamic twist helps mobilize the back, engage the obliques, and release tension from the midsection.

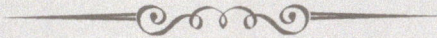

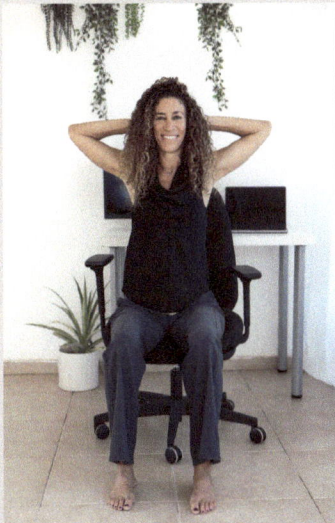

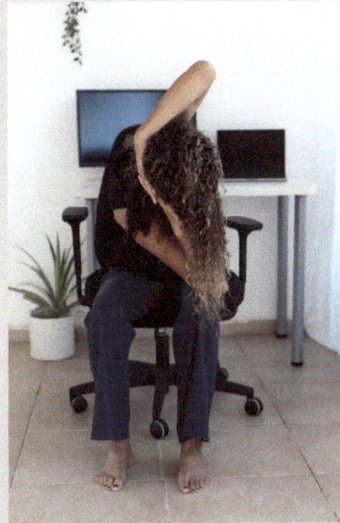

Exercise 4: Seated Side Bend

Sit tall with your feet grounded and spine lengthened. Place your right hand on the chair's arm rest or the outer side of the chair for support. Inhale and bring your left arm up and over, reaching toward the right side as you bend gently from the waist.
Keep both sit bones anchored and avoid collapsing forward—aim to open through the side body. Feel the stretch from your hip up through your ribs and into your arm. Hold for a few breaths, smile, then return to center and repeat on the other side*.

This movement releases tension in the lower back, ribs, and waist, and encourages deeper breathing.

*Note: Your gaze while in the pose can be forward, up or down - depends what feels comfortable for your neck at that moment. See variation examples in the photos.

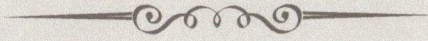

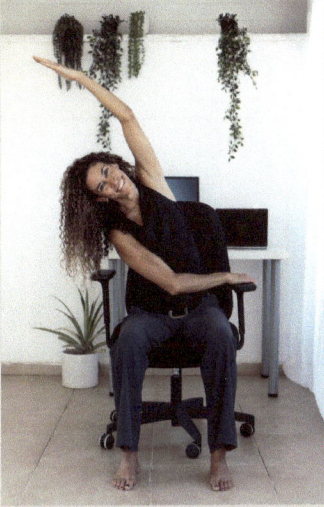
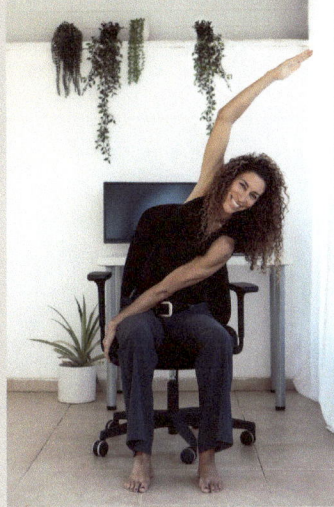

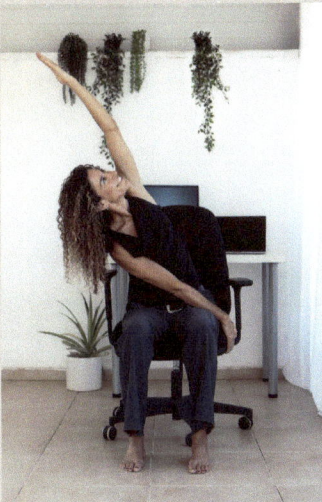
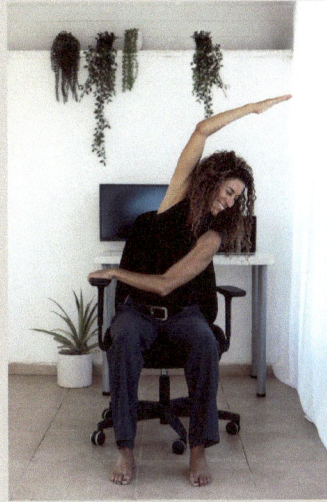

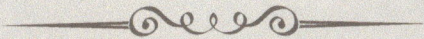

Exercise 5: Seated Forward Fold

 Sit near the edge of your chair with feet hip-width apart and firmly planted. Inhale to sit up tall and lengthen the spine. As you exhale, hinge at the hips and fold forward, letting your torso rest over your thighs.
Start by lengthening your arms and extend the spine before you allow your head, neck, and arms to relax fully—hands can dangle, rest on the floor or hug the legs.

It is recommended to close the eyes. Breathe deeply and stay for several slow breaths.
To come back up, press into your feet and slowly roll up, stacking the spine one vertebra at a time.

This fold gently stretches the back, hips, and hamstrings, while calming the nervous system and relieving spinal compression.

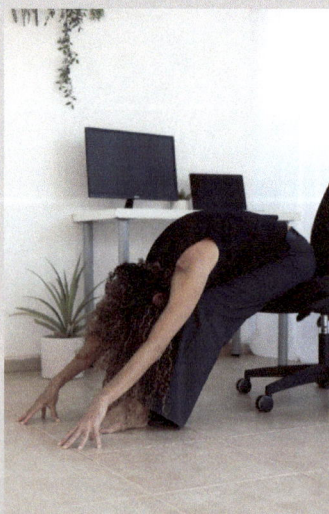

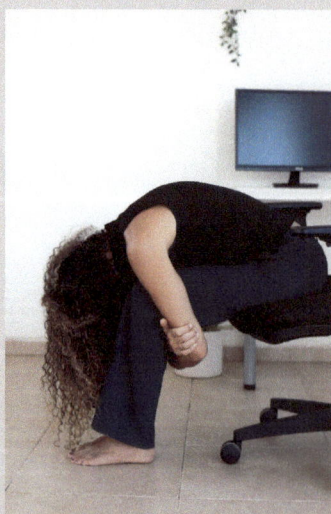

7

HIPS

The hips are a central hub in the body, connecting the upper and lower halves and supporting almost every movement we make - walking, sitting, standing, bending.

When the hips are tight or restricted, the body compensates elsewhere, often leading to strain in the lower back, knees, or even shoulders.

Regular hip movement and stretching help maintain mobility, improve posture, and support a healthy spine.
Releasing tension in the hips also increases circulation, reduces stiffness, and creates a sense of ease in the whole body.

For anyone sitting for long periods or doing repetitive movements, keeping the hips open and mobile is key to preventing pain and preserving long-term joint health.

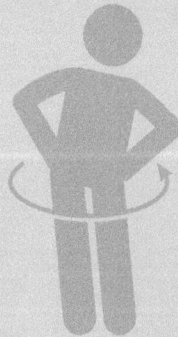

Exercise 1: Seated Marching

Sit upright at the edge of a chair with feet flat on the floor and core engaged. On an inhale, lift your right knee toward your chest - just as high as is comfortable - engaging the hip flexors. Exhale to lower it back down with control. Repeat on the left side.

 Continue alternating legs in a smooth, rhythmic motion for 10–12 repetitions each side Keep the spine long and avoid leaning back. Your arms can rest on the chair or you can stretch them forward.

This movement helps activate and mobilize the hip flexors, improving circulation, coordination, and strength - especially helpful after long periods of sitting when these muscles tend to shorten and tighten.

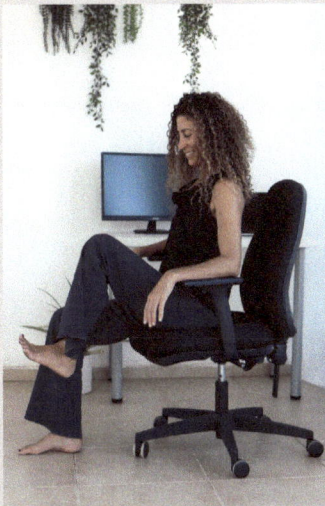

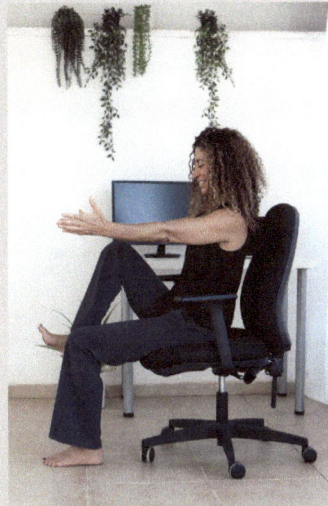

Exercise 2: Seated Figure Four Stretch

Sit tall on your chair with both feet flat on the ground. Lift your right foot and place your right ankle across your left thigh, just above the knee - creating a "figure four" shape. Flex the right foot to protect the knee joint.
Sit up tall as you inhale, and as you exhale, gently hinge forward at the hips to deepen the stretch*.

You should feel a stretch in the outer hip and glute of the lifted leg. Hold for 5–8 breaths (you can close your eyes and smile), then slowly switch sides.

This stretch is excellent for releasing deep hip tension, especially from long periods of sitting.

*Note: Only deepen the stretch if there is no tension or pain in the knee.

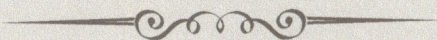

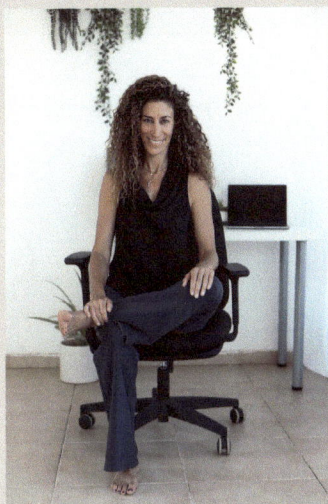
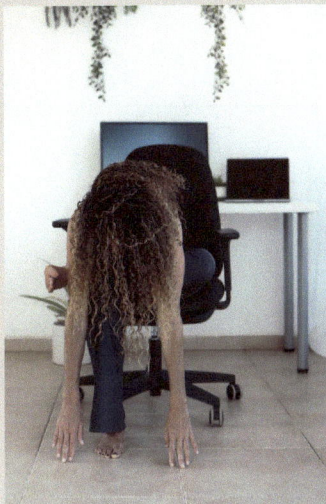

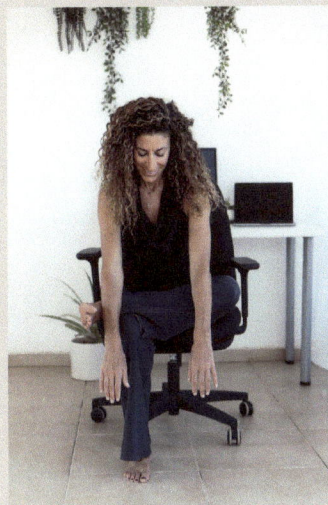
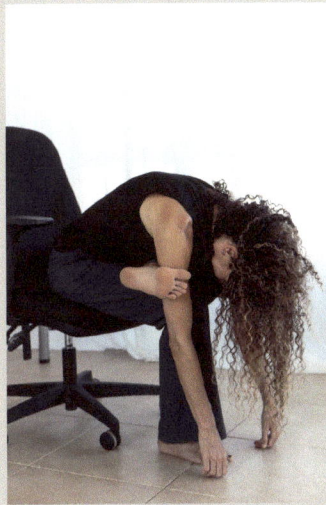

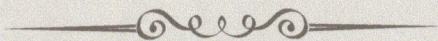

Optional - Add a twist

To add a gentle spinal twist, bring your outer arm across to press against the inside of your foot, while your upper arm reaches upward. Press gently into the foot to help deepen the twist.
Your gaze can be upward or forward - whichever feels most comfortable for your neck.

Continue to breathe deeply, allowing each breath to release the spine and the hips (don't forget to smile).

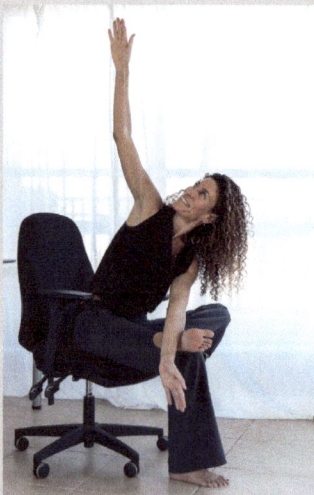

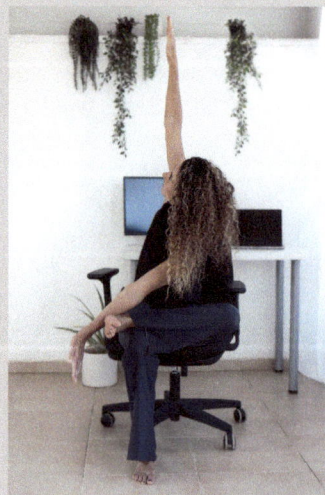

8

ANKLES&FEET

Our feet and ankles are the foundation of our posture and movement - supporting us throughout the day, especially when we sit or stand for long periods. Yet, they're often overlooked in desk-based routines. Stiffness or reduced mobility in these joints can impact circulation, balance, and even the alignment of the knees, hips, and spine.

Incorporating gentle Yoga-inspired movements helps stimulate blood flow, improve joint mobility, and release tension built up from inactivity.

These simple exercises can awaken your awareness of the ground beneath you, boost energy, and bring a refreshing sense of lightness from the ground up.

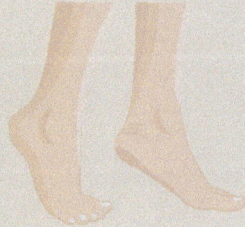

Exercise 1: Toe Lifts & Spreads

This is our opportunity to strengthen the foot muscles, improve circulation, and relieve tension from prolonged sitting. If you are wearing shoes, this is the time to take them off.

Sit tall on your chair with both feet flat on the floor, hip-width apart. Keep your heels grounded and slowly lift all ten toes up. Try to spread your toes away from each other as much as possible - like a fan. Hold for 3 breaths, then slowly lower the toes back down.

Repeat for 5–8 rounds. Try alternating lifting just the big toe while keeping the others down, and vice versa, to awaken fine motor control.

Exercise 2: Ankle Circles

Here is an easy way to improve range of motion in the ankles, stimulate blood flow, prevent stiffness and swelling (and you can keep your shoes on for this one).

Sit upright on your chair, feet a little forward from the base of the chair. Lift your right foot a few centimeters off the floor, keeping your knee bent and steady. Begin to circle your ankle clockwise - slow and controlled - for about 5–8 circles.
Then switch to counter-clockwise for the same number of circles.
Repeat with the left ankle.

Imagine drawing big circles with your toes while keeping the rest of the leg relaxed and still. Smile.

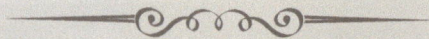

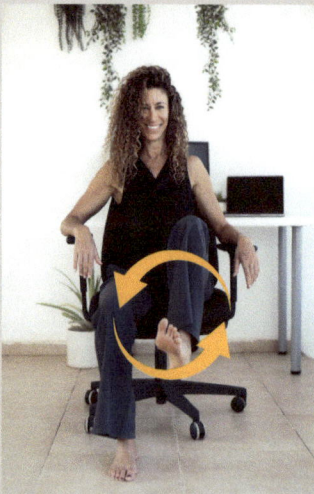

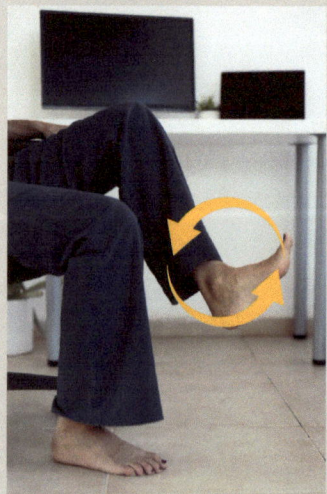

Exercise 3: Ankle Pumps and core stability

Let's get these calf muscles working so that we build strength in the front and back of the lower leg, supporting ankle stability and circulation. This in turn will improve our control and resilience in the ankle joint.

Sit tall on your chair with both feet flat on the floor. Lift your right leg and extend it forward. Flex your foot and make sure you are not collapsing in your lower back. Point your toes forward (like pressing a gas pedal), then flex them back toward your face.

Move slowly and deliberately, repeat 10–15 times, then switch to the other leg. Whenever you feel it is too much, you can lower your leg and rest. Don't forget to smile.

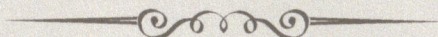

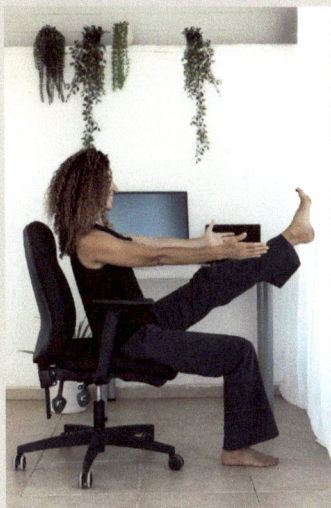

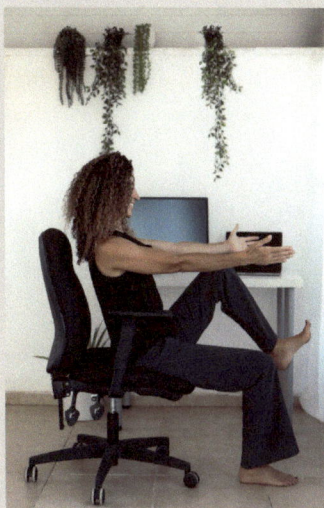

Exercise 4: Ankle Stretch with Foot Cross

Now that we have worked the joints and supportive muscles, it is time to gently stretch the ankle, top of the foot, and shin. This exercise will help release tension from the foot and ankle, improve flexibility and prevent discomfort from static sitting.

Sit upright and cross your right ankle over your left thigh, letting the foot rest gently. Hold your right ankle with your left hand, and gently press down on the top of your right foot with your right hand, pointing the toes downward slightly. You should feel a stretch across the front of the ankle and top of the foot. Hold for 3–5 breaths, then switch sides.

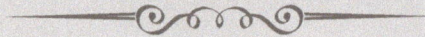

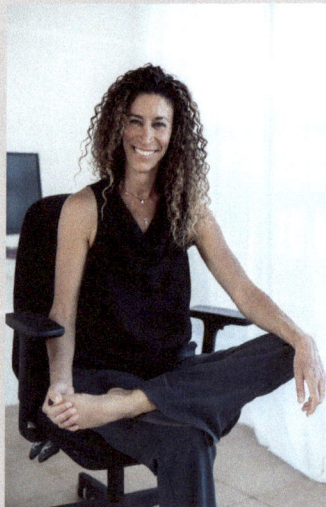

Optional - Foot massage

After the stretch, take this opportunity to gently massage your foot, applying light pressure to any areas that need your attention.

Use your thumb to apply pressure and explore the sensations in your feet.

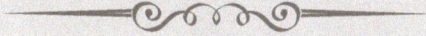

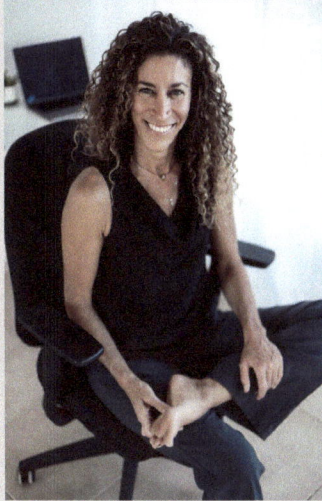

9
CALMING THE MIND

In today's fast-paced world, our minds are constantly stimulated - pinging from email to app, screen to screen. While our bodies sit still, our thoughts rarely do. This ongoing mental chatter can lead to stress, fatigue, and a sense of disconnection - both from ourselves and the present moment.

This chapter invites you to pause. To give your mind a well-deserved break from analysis, problem-solving, and scrolling. We do this by bringing awareness to something beautifully simple and always available - the breath.

Practising breath-focused meditation, even for just a few minutes a day, helps shift the nervous system from "fight or flight" into a state of calm. Over time, meditation becomes a powerful tool to:
- Reduce stress and anxiety
- Improve focus and emotional clarity
- Support restful sleep
- Enhance resilience and overall well-being

Like training a muscle, the more consistently you practice, the easier it becomes to return to a place of stillness - even in the midst of a busy workday. This is not about stopping your thoughts. It's about anchoring your awareness in the present and giving your mind the space it needs to breathe.

Exercise 1: One-Minute Breath Focus

Purpose: A simple, accessible meditation to calm the nervous system, anchor attention, and reduce mental fatigue.

Sit comfortably on your chair, feet grounded and hands resting gently on your thighs or in your lap. Soften your shoulders and close your eyes, or keep your gaze low and unfocused. Begin by taking a gentle breath in through your nose and exhale slowly through your nose.

Bring your full attention to the sensation of breathing - notice the rise and fall of your chest, the air passing through your nostrils, or the subtle movement in your belly. If your mind wanders (and it will), gently return your focus to the breath - again and again, without judgment. Continue this for one minute, or as long as it feels good.

Optional Anchor:
Silently say "in" as you breathe in and "out" as you breathe out.
This helps steady the mind.

Exercise 2: Three-Minutes Body Scan

Purpose: Brings awareness to the body, reduces tension, and grounds the mind in the present.

Sit comfortably, feet on the floor, hands resting on your lap. Gently close your eyes or soften your gaze. Take a deep breath in, and as you exhale, allow your body to settle.
Begin by bringing your awareness to the crown of your head. Notice any sensations or lack thereof. No need to change anything - just observe.

Slowly move your attention downward: to your forehead, jaw, neck and shoulders. Let each area soften as you notice it.
Continue scanning down your arms, chest, back, and abdomen.
Move through the hips, thighs, knees, lower legs, and finally into your feet.

If your mind wanders, gently bring it back to wherever you left off. End with one deep breath and open your eyes gently when you are ready.

Exercise 3: Loving-Kindness Meditation

Whenever you need it during your day -
Beginning, middle or end, this practice
cultivates compassion, emotional balance, and
a deeper connection with others.

Sit comfortably and bring one or both hands to
your heart if that feels good. Take a few gentle
breaths to settle. Silently repeat these phrases,
first directing them toward yourself:
May I be safe
May I be healthy
May I be at ease
May I be happy

Now bring someone to mind whom you care
about. Repeat:
May you be safe
May you be healthy
May you be at ease
May you be happy

If you'd like, extend this to a neutral person, or
even someone you find challenging.

When practising loving-kindness meditation, it is important to go slowly and connect with the meaning behind the words. If emotions arise, allow them.

This practice helps us to build empathy and emotional resilience, support healthy relationships and teamwork, reduces self-criticism and boosts positive emotion.

Imagine a world in which this was a daily practice by everyone.

"Be the change you want to see in the world"

— Mahatma Gandhi

Thank you

To the companies who welcomed Yoga into the workday:
Thank you for believing in the importance of well-being, and for allowing the space to bring presence and movement into your employees' lives.

To my friends, colleagues, and students who offered thoughtful feedback, shared their experience, and supported this vision:
Your encouragement means more than words can express.

To the talented photographer Aviya Cohen for capturing the postures.

May this little guide bring ease, strength, and stillness - one breath at a time.

With gratitude,
Shani

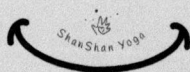

ShanShan Yoga

ShanShan Yoga

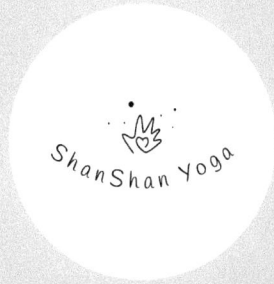

Find the joy within

"Sometimes your joy is the source of your smile, but sometimes your smile can be the source of your joy."

— Thich Nhat Hanh

www.ingramcontent.com/pod-product-compliance
Lightning Source LLC
Chambersburg PA
CBHW041308020426
42333CB00001B/13